DEMENTIA

A *Handbook* for *Long-Term Care* Activities Staff

Frosini Rubertino, RN, C-NE, CDONA/LTC, CPRA

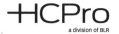

Dementia Care: A Handbook for Long-Term Care Activities Staff is published by HCPro, a division of BLR.

Copyright © 2014 HCPro, a division of BLR.

All rights reserved. Printed in the United States of America.   5 4 3 2 1

ISBN: 978-1-55645-138-6

No part of this publication may be reproduced, in any form or by any means, without prior written consent of HCPro, or the Copyright Clearance Center (978-750-8400). Please notify us immediately if you have received an unauthorized copy.

HCPro provides information resources for the healthcare industry.

HCPro is not affiliated in any way with The Joint Commission, which owns the JCAHO and Joint Commission trademarks.

Frosini Rubertino, RN, BSN, Author
Olivia MacDonald, Managing Editor
Adrienne Trivers, Product Manager
Erin Callahan, Senior Director, Product
Elizabeth Petersen, Vice President
Matt Sharpe, Production Supervisor
Vincent Skyers, Design Manager
Vicki McMahan, Sr. Graphic Designer
Jason Gregory, Layout/Graphic Design
Mike King, Cover Designer

Advice given is general. Readers should consult professional counsel for specific legal, ethical, or clinical questions.

Arrangements can be made for quantity discounts. For more information, contact:

HCPro
75 Sylvan Street, Suite A-101
Danvers, MA 01923
Telephone: 800-650-6787 or 781-639-1872
Fax: 800-639-8511
Email: *customerservice@hcpro.com*

Visit HCPro online at: *www.hcpro.com* and *www.hcmarketplace.com*

Contents

About the Author v
Foreword vii
Chapter 1: Dementia Care in Long-Term Care 1
Chapter 2: Understanding Dementia and Person-Centered Care 9
Chapter 3: Building an Interdisciplinary Dementia Care Team 19
Chapter 4: Conditions That Impact Cognitive Functioning 25
Chapter 5: Assessment of Behavioral Conditions 29
Chapter 6: Non-Pharmacological Approaches to Managing Dementia Behaviors 35
Chapter 7: Pharmacological Approaches to Managing Dementia Behaviors 41
Chapter 8: Monitoring Outcomes of Approaches 47
Chapter 9: Dementia Care and Activities Staff 51
Dementia Care Resources 57

About the Author

Frosini Rubertino, RN, BSN, is a regulatory specialist with over 25 years of experience in the healthcare industry. She is the author of *The QIS Mock Survey Guide* (HCPro); *The Medicare Billing Manual for Long-Term Care* (HCPro); and *Carmelina: Essential Nursing Systems for Long-Term Care* (TrainingInMotion.org).

As the founder of TrainingInMotion.org and an HCPro Boot Camps™ instructor, she is a nationally recognized instructor and speaker, advising long-term care organizations in regulatory compliance and how to maintain excellence in their respective roles.

She is also a contributor to numerous publications including *PPS Alert for Long-Term Care, Billing Alert for Long-Term Care,* and the author of several published articles in *Provider Magazine* and *The Eden Alternative*®. She is often a featured speaker regarding clinical systems, culture change, performance improvement, and Medicare for state and private organizations across the country.

Foreword

Dementia. It can happen to anyone. It has no allegiance to any one culture, gender, or geographic location. The World Health Organization (WHO) reports there is an estimated 35.6 million people living with dementia worldwide. That number is expected to double by 2030 and is likely to triple by 2050. The Alzheimer's Association reports Alzheimer's-type dementia as the sixth-leading cause of death in the United States. Approximately 200,000 individuals who are younger than 65 years old are stricken with the disease.

WHO dementia facts
1. Dementia is not a normal part of aging
2. 35.6 million people live with dementia worldwide
3. A new case of dementia is diagnosed every four seconds around the world
4. The economic impact of caring for people with dementia in the United States is $604 billion
5. Dementia caregivers experience a high level of stress

6. Early diagnosis can improve the quality of life for people with dementia
7. Many people with dementia are discriminated against through the use of physical and chemical restraints
8. More awareness and advocacy for dementia care is needed to improve the quality of life for people with dementia
9. More research is needed to develop new and more effective interventions and treatments
10. Dementia is a public health priority, in which the public needs more education about it to improve attitudes and understanding of the disease

Dementia care is an interdisciplinary collaborative approach. Key elements of dementia care include staff education, environmental adaptations, provisions for recognizing and meeting spiritual and psychological needs, the implementation of a social model of care that allows the resident to perform valued activities and to participate in their own care to the full extent of their capabilities, avoiding unnecessary antipsychotic use, and providing support for family and caregivers. The interdisciplinary collaborative approach includes not only each department in the long-term care facility, but across the continuum of care, provider to provider. As the disease progresses, so should our approach to accommodate ongoing quality of life for people with dementia. It's a journey of caring enough to do the right thing and caring enough to do more.

Chapter 1: Dementia Care in Long-Term Care

Dementia care in long-term care continues to evolve, bringing with it new and higher expectations to improve quality of life and quality of care. There have been several significant strides and events toward the goal of improving how we manage our dementia care practices; however, a "gold standard" has yet to be established and because of this, we are left with assembling information from a variety of resources to provide quality dementia care. If we are resourceful and open-minded, we can begin to develop our facility's own gold-standard goal for dementia care that includes meeting needs beyond the activities of daily living, and into a more holistic person-centered framework of services. This manual will help you accomplish this goal.

The American Medical Directors Association (AMDA), dedicated to long-term care medicine, published clinical practice guidelines *(Dementia in the Long Term Care Setting – Clinical Practice Guideline)* for dementia care in nursing homes. The AMDA works closely with House and Senate leaders to address the use of antipsychotics in nursing homes, and its vice president has testified at the Senate Special Committee on Aging hearing titled, "Overprescribed: The Human and Taxpayers' Costs of Antipsychotics in Nursing Homes" (U.S. Senate, Special Committee on Aging, Washington, D.C., November 30, 2011). The hearing examined the use of antipsychotics among nursing home residents with dementia despite the U.S. Food and Drug Administration's black box warnings for use, and discussed the need for safe and effective alternatives, citing increased risk of death when antipsychotics are used to treat the elderly who do not have a diagnosis of psychosis. An interdisciplinary approach to person-centered care was stressed for behavior management, while decreasing the use of unnecessary medication.

From a regulatory perspective, in March 2010 Congress passed the Patient Protection and Affordable Care Act (PPACA), often referred to as the Affordable Care Act (ACA), with Part III Section 6121 amending the Social Security Act, Sections 1829 and 1919, that are requirements to include initial and ongoing dementia management training and abuse prevention training for nursing assistants.

> *A(i) requirements for the approval of nurse aide training and competency evaluation programs, including requirements relating to (I) the areas to be covered in such a program (including at least basic nursing skills, personal care skills, recognition of mental health and social service needs, care of cognitively impaired residents, basic restorative services, and residents' rights) and content of the curriculum (including, in the case of initial training and, if the Secretary determines appropriate, in the case of ongoing training, dementia management training, and patient abuse prevention training, (II) minimum hours of initial and ongoing*

> *training and retraining (including not less than 75 hours in the case of initial training), (III) qualifications of instructors, and (IV) procedures for determination of competency.*

In 2011, the Office of Inspector General (OIG) released a report, which indicated 83% of nursing home residents did not have a proper diagnosis to justify the use of their antipsychotic medication. AMDA now includes a free interactive course to its members aimed at decreasing inappropriate antipsychotic use in persons with dementia.

In 2012, the Centers for Medicare & Medicaid Services (CMS) launched the National Partnership to Improve Dementia Care, now referred to as Partnership to Improve Dementia Care in Nursing Homes. An important aspect of this initiative is to reduce the unnecessary use of antipsychotics. Issues such as pain management, caregiver stress, and decision-making on dementia care interventions also remain areas of concern. A pilot project is underway to examine the process of dementia care in nursing homes and to take a closer look at the prescribing of antipsychotics. Among other providers, advocacy groups and caregivers, the AMDA also joined this partnership.

From a survey perspective, the CMS Center for Clinical Standards and Quality/Survey & Certification Group released a memorandum in May 2013 conveying clarifications for the survey process regarding dementia care and unnecessary drug use. Another memorandum was released in April 2014 regarding a focused survey process to assess dementia care and outlines five fundamental principles of dementia care:

1. **Person–Centered Care.** CMS requires nursing homes to provide a supportive environment that promotes comfort and recognizes individual needs and preferences.

2. **Quality and Quantity of Staff.** The nursing home must provide staff, both in terms of quantity (direct care as well as supervisory staff) and quality, to meet the needs of the residents as determined by resident assessments and individual plans of care.

3. **Thorough Evaluation of New or Worsening Behaviors.** Residents who exhibit new or worsening behavioral or psychological symptoms of dementia (BPSD) should have an evaluation by the interdisciplinary team, including the physician, in order to identify and address treatable medical, physical, emotional, psychiatric, psychological, functional, social, and environmental factors that may be contributing to behaviors.

4. **Individualized Approaches to Care.** Current guidelines from the United States, United Kingdom, Canada, and other countries recommend the use of individualized approaches as a first-line intervention (except in documented emergency situations or if clinically contraindicated) for BPSD. Utilizing a consistent process that focuses on a resident's individual needs and tries to understand behavior as a form of communication may help to reduce behavioral expressions of distress in some residents.

5. **Critical Thinking Related to Antipsychotic Drug Use.** In certain cases, residents may benefit from the use of medications. The resident should only be given medication if clinically indicated and as necessary to treat a specific condition and target symptoms as diagnosed and documented in the record. Residents who use antipsychotic drugs must receive gradual dose reductions and behavioral interventions, unless clinically contraindicated, in an effort to discontinue these drugs.

Survey agencies will use, at a minimum, regulation F309 (Quality of Care) and F329 (Unnecessary Drugs) to investigate services for a resident with dementia. In May 2013, CMS issued a memorandum, 13-35-NH, for the *State Operations Manual* regarding dementia care. The update states that during the Entrance Conference in Task 2 of the traditional survey process, surveyors will ask for "a list of names of residents who have a diagnosis of dementia and who are receiving, have received, or presently have PRN orders for antipsychotic medications over the past 30 days." The administrator or the director of nursing will be asked to "describe how the facility provides individualized care and services for residents with dementia and to provide policies related to the use of antipsychotic medication in residents with dementia." In the Quality Indicator Survey process, surveyors will not necessarily ask for information regarding those with dementia and antipsychotic use since their survey software will automatically identify the required survey sample. Included in the memorandum is a "Resident with Dementia Checklist" that may be used to guide the investigation for both survey processes that includes assessment and underlying cause identification, care planning, implementation of the care plan, care plan revision, monitoring, follow-up, and quality assessment and assurance. This checklist can be found at the end of the *State Operations Manual* updates in the "SURVEY AND CERTIFICATION MEMORANDUM, S&C: 13-35-NH" issued May 24, 2013.

F309 Quality of Care
Regulatory language:
Each resident must receive and the facility must provide the necessary care and services to attain or maintain the highest practicable physical, mental, and psychosocial well-being, in accordance with the comprehensive assessment and plan of care.

The intent of F309:

The facility must ensure that the resident obtains optimal improvement or does not deteriorate within the limits of a resident's right to refuse treatment, and within the limits of recognized pathology and the normal aging process.

F329 Unnecessary Drugs

Regulatory language:

1. General. Each resident's drug regimen must be free from unnecessary drugs. An unnecessary drug is any drug when used:
    i. In excessive dose (including duplicate therapy); or
    ii. For excessive duration; or
    iii. Without adequate monitoring; or
    iv. Without adequate indications for its use; or
    v. In the presence of adverse consequences which indicate the dose should be reduced or discontinued; or
    vi. Any combinations of the reasons above.

2. Antipsychotic Drugs. Based on a comprehensive assessment of a resident, the facility must ensure that:
    i. Residents who have not used antipsychotic drugs are not given these drugs unless antipsychotic drug therapy is necessary to treat a specific condition as diagnosed and documented in the clinical record; and
    ii. Residents who use antipsychotic drugs receive gradual dose reductions, and behavioral interventions, unless clinically contraindicated, in an effort to discontinue these drugs.

The intent of F329:

The intent of this requirement is that each resident's entire drug/medication regimen be managed and monitored to achieve the following goals:

- The medication regimen helps promote or maintain the resident's highest practicable mental, physical, and psychosocial well-being, as identified by the resident and/or representative(s) in collaboration with the attending physician and facility staff;
- Each resident receives only those medications, in doses and for the duration clinically indicated to treat the resident's assessed condition(s);
- Non-pharmacological interventions (such as behavioral interventions) are considered and used when indicated, instead of, or in addition to, medication;
- Clinically significant adverse consequences are minimized; and
- The potential contribution of the medication regimen to an unanticipated decline or newly emerging or worsening symptom is recognized and evaluated, and the regimen is modified when appropriate.

Together, the PPACA, the CMS Partnership, AMDA, and the surveyor guidance will significantly expand the scope of quality dementia care expectations in nursing homes across America, focusing on staff education and accountability for person-centered approaches to meet the care needs of those with dementia. If we work as an advocate and as a collaborative interdisciplinary team, utilizing the resources available to us, we can develop a gold standard of dementia care across the entire continuum of care that will change the culture of aging in our country and hopefully influence dementia care for the 35.6 million individuals around the world who are diagnosed with dementia.

Chapter 2: Understanding Dementia and Person-Centered Care

The term *dementia* is used to describe a group of disorders that affect daily functioning. It is not a specific disease, but is considered an umbrella term for the group of disorders with symptoms that affect physical, social, and cognitive function. While there are several types of dementia, Alzheimer's disease is the most common type of progressive irreversible dementia. Other irreversible dementias include vascular dementia, mixed dementia, Parkinson's disease, and Lewy body (Table 2.1). Less common are Frontotemporal, Huntington's, Wernicke-Korsakoff syndrome, Creutzfeldt-Jakob disease, and AIDS-related dementia.

Table 2.1: Description of irreversible dementias

Alzheimer's	The most common type of dementia.
	Accounts for 60%–80% of all dementias.
	Brain cells degenerate and die, causing memory and mental function declines.
Vascular	Caused by impaired blood flow to the brain, such as after a stroke from a blood clot or hemorrhage.
	May also be a result of other conditions, including the brain being deprived of oxygen due to vascular disease, head injuries, or heart attack.
	High cholesterol, smoking, and high blood pressure significantly increase the chances of vascular dementia.
Mixed	Having symptoms of more than one type of dementia. For example, a combination of Alzheimer's dementia and vascular dementia.
Lewy Body	May result in muscle rigidity, slow movement, tremors, and hallucinations.
	May also go back and forth from moments of clarity to moments of confusion.
	Often misdiagnosed as Parkinson's disease due to the appearance of tremors, or Alzheimer's disease due to the memory loss.

Table 2.1: Description of irreversible dementias (cont.)

Parkinson's	Approximately 50% of those with Parkinson's disease may experience dementia.
	May begin with tremors, but progresses to speech problems such as mumbling.
	Face often appears to have no facial expression.
	Arms may not swing when walking.
Frontotemporal	Affects frontal and temporal lobes of the brain.
	Symptoms will affect personality, behavior, and language.
Huntington's	Will include behavioral changes and abnormal movements of the face and extremities.
	May experience difficulty swallowing and speech impairment.
Wernicke-Korsakoff	This is a degenerative brain disorder.
	Caused by lack of vitamin B1, alcohol abuse, prolonged vomiting, or side effects of chemotherapy.
Creutzfeldt-Jakob	Rare, degenerative, and fatal.
	Progresses quickly leading to death.
AIDS-related	Inability to concentrate with poor short-term memory.
	May include motor dysfunction and behavioral changes.

The Effects of Dementia on Daily Life

Dementia is not a normal part of aging, but is most common after the age of 65. More and more, we are seeing early onset in individuals who are in age groups from 30 to 50. The following areas may be compromised at different levels for each resident depending on the progression of his or her specific type of dementia:

Memory	Unable to remember recent or long-term events
Concentration	Unable to stay focused on the task
Orientation	Do not know who they are, what they are doing, what time or day it is, where they are
Language	Experiencing difficulty communicating or making their needs known, understanding what others are saying
Visuospatial	Cannot make sense of surroundings and objects, may not be able to find own room, running into furniture
Judgment	Makes poor safety decisions
Sequencing	Unable to do things in a logical order
Patience	Cannot remain calm in an environment that is confusing to them
Physical function	At risk of injury and nutritional deficiency due to memory loss, impaired mobility, unidentified pain, and self-care deficits
Social	Experiences impaired relationships with family and caregivers
Emotional	May experience outbursts, crying, depression, apathy, yelling, or anxiety
Other	Wandering unsafely, inability to make healthcare decisions or financial decisions

How Does Dementia Influence Person-Centered Care?

Each symptom intervention must be targeted to the individual needs of each resident. Not all residents with dementia have the same needs. Personalities, culture, social history, physical limitations, type of dementia, level of education, and severity of dementia symptoms are all factors requiring consideration for an effective dementia care

Chapter 2: Understanding Dementia and Person-Centered Care

program and will influence how an individual reacts in a variety of life situations.

Resultant behaviors in an individual with dementia may be a product of frustration, loneliness, boredom, fear, helplessness, or confusion. Thus, the focus of dementia care needs to be person-centered and holistic. The following person-centered care approach case studies illustrate the various approaches for each individual.

Name/Age:	Mrs. Kramer 84 years old
Diagnosis:	Alzheimer's dementia, high blood pressure, and diabetes
Prior history	She enjoyed vegetable gardening and caring for her rose bushes.
Trigger	No opportunity to go outside since admitted to nursing home.
Resultant behavior	Agitation during idle time spent going to indoor activities in facility.
Person-centered care approach	Provide resident the ability to go outside, participate in gardening, if available.

Name/Age:	Mr. Smith/76 years old
Diagnosis:	Mixed Dementia
Prior history	Loves to read.
Trigger	Doesn't have books in room. Facility does not have a library.
Resultant behavior	Frustrated by lack of ability to read.
Person-centered care approach	Provide resident the ability to go outside, participate in gardening, if available. Read to resident one-on-one when staff sees he is beginning to become frustrated.

Name/Age:	Mrs. Benedict/69 years old
Diagnosis:	Alzheimer's dementia, early stages
Prior history	Owned a catering business, enjoyed baking.
Trigger	Most activities provided are too confusing to follow, so she's avoiding them.
Resultant behavior	Confusion and helplessness at not being able to follow/ remember steps to provided activities.
Person-centered care approach	Include her in a baking activity, reminding her each step of the way of the ingredients and directions on preparation.

Name/Age:	Mr. Silverton/80 years old
Diagnosis:	Alzheimer's dementia
Prior history	Career construction foreman, traveled between sites overseeing workers.
Trigger	Needs to keep busy. Does not like boredom.
Resultant behavior	Wanders in and out of rooms, frequently attempts to leave facility.
Person-centered care approach	His behaviors may best be managed by determining what times he begins to wander and include him in a small group activity with adequate supervision.

Chapter 2: Understanding Dementia and Person-Centered Care

Name/Age: Mrs. Perry/74 years old	
Diagnosis: Lewy body dementia.	
Prior history	Does not speak fluent English. Lived with her daughter who interpreted conversations for her.
Trigger	Wants to understand what people are saying.
Resultant behavior	She becomes frustrated during dressing, resulting in combative behavior when staff attempts to complete the entire dressing task for her.
Person-centered care approach	Her behaviors may best be managed by allowing her to participate in her care, breaking the task of dressing down to smaller tasks, and giving her time to complete each step.

Name/Age: Mr. Cunningham/82 years old	
Diagnosis: Mixed dementia.	
Prior history	Retired accountant.
Trigger	His osteoarthritis and rheumatoid arthritis. Requires frequent administration of PRN pain medication throughout day. Gets frustrated when he attempts to write due to pain in his fingers.
Resultant behavior	He becomes agitated when staff approaches him for transferring and positioning. Has stopped participating in activities.
Person-centered care approach	Managing his pain symptoms with a program that anticipates the pain, rather than responding to it when he already hurts, may help improve his response to caregiving.

Name/Age:	Mrs. Lentz/78 years old
Diagnosis:	Vascular dementia
Prior history	Was previously able to be independent with her healthcare decisions. Minimal chronic conditions.
Trigger	Documentation in the medical record indicates she has not had her ears examined for over three years. She is having difficulty hearing.
Resultant behavior	Becomes frustrated and eventually agitated when staff attempts to verbally interact with her.
Person-centered care approach	A simple earwax removal procedure by the physician may unblock her ears and help her hear what staff is saying to her, resulting in fewer episodes of frustration and agitation.

Name/Age:	Mr. Carlton/81 years old
Diagnosis:	Parkinson's dementia, and benign prostatic hypertrophy (BPH), and congestive heart failure.
Prior history	Urinary urgency from BPH, bathroom door was within 6 feet of bed at home. Takes a diuretic at 7 a.m. each morning.
Trigger	He wanders in and out of rooms after breakfast each day.
Resultant behavior	When he is found in other resident rooms, he is often incontinent. He is most likely attempting to find a bathroom.
Person-centered care approach	Anticipating his toileting needs, after a toileting diary is completed and implementing a prompted toileting plan, may decrease the wandering.

Name/Age: Mrs. Lampin/83 years old	
Diagnosis: Parkinson's dementia.	
Prior history	Former night shift nurse supervisor.
Trigger	Accustomed to napping after breakfast and after lunch. However, she is often left up in her wheelchair at those times.
Resultant behavior	She becomes uncooperative and agitated with staff during those times of the day. Has difficulty falling asleep at night.
Person-centered care approach	Accommodating her naps may eliminate those behaviors, or accommodate her when she chooses to stay awake at night.

In many cases, behavior may be a response to caregiver behaviors and actions. Consider how a resident may respond to the following situations:

- Scheduling showers for a resident who previously took only baths
- Beginning a task without first informing the resident what you are going to do
- Physically blocking a resident who is wandering
- Using the word "no" to stop a resident from doing something
- Waking residents up early in the morning when they may prefer to sleep in later
- High noise levels and bright lights
- Not interacting with the resident during care delivery
- Staff moving too quickly through the task, hurrying the resident

Person-centered care requires the education of staff, residents, and families, with substantial coordination between interdisciplinary team members, to create alternative modalities to possible and potential triggers of behaviors.

In addition to education, implementing person-centered care approaches may require staffing levels that are beyond your state requirements. Each state has minimum staffing requirements based on resident-to-staff ratios, based on total census, or some other methodology. However, this does not exclude the facility from providing sufficient staffing to meet the needs of the residents, especially those with dementia. In fact, F353: Nursing Services, addresses sufficient staffing with the intent to ensure sufficient qualified nursing staff is available on a daily basis to meet the care needs of each resident in an environment that will enhance quality of life. This regulatory F-tag specifically states:

> *The facility must have sufficient nursing staff to provide nursing and related services to attain or maintain the highest practicable physical, mental, and psychosocial well-being of each resident, as determined by resident assessments and individual plans of care.*

From education to staffing, it will take time to develop a culture of person-centered care approaches for your facility. It is best to begin with the individuals with the most behaviors or distress. You will need to assemble and educate a dementia care team that will work collaboratively with other disciplines and the family to identify the root cause of the behavior and implement interventions to target those causes. Keep in mind that all behavior is purposeful. Find out what the resident is trying to do, why he or she is trying to do it, and then figure out how to meet that need.

Chapter 3: Building an Interdisciplinary Dementia Care Team

Dementia care requires the transition from a multidisciplinary to an interdisciplinary care team approach. A multidisciplinary approach is defined as being non-integrative, while an interdisciplinary approach crosses the boundaries of each discipline. The key component that differentiates these two approaches is collaboration. No one discipline can possess the sole knowledge or expertise to address a problem. The combined contribution is much greater than any one discipline can offer. Integrating the knowledge of each discipline while harmonizing and transcending the traditional boundaries will move us close to an interdisciplinary approach. The comparative chart below demonstrates the differences between the two approaches (Table 3.1).

Table 3.1: Multidisciplinary vs. interdisciplinary

Multidisciplinary team members	Interdisciplinary team members
Each discipline retains its own ideas on interventions without input from other disciplines.	Crosses boundaries of each discipline, with respectful communication.
Shares knowledge but stays within their boundaries.	Analyzes and harmonizes links between disciplines.
Little direct communication, working parallel with each other.	Engaged and learn from each other; the entire team assumes responsibility for care.
Several disciplines generally meet without the resident to discuss interventions for a problem.	Integrates all disciplines into a single consultation, including the resident or his or her representative, yielding a person-centered approach.
Protects traditional boundaries.	Transcends traditional boundaries.
Department head–centered.	Patient-centered.
May result in duplication of interventions without communication of outcomes.	Lack of duplication of interventions with shared communication of outcomes.
Lack of coordination leads to poor outcomes.	Coordination of care improves outcomes.

Transitioning to an Interdisciplinary Approach

A successful transition from multidisciplinary to interdisciplinary begins with a team facilitator who understands the process of team building and fosters each discipline's participation, while each team member must learn to respect and value each other's contributions to the ultimate goal. Team members will ultimately experience professional satisfaction in an innovative environment, gaining new skills and knowledge along the way. Staff time and resources will be utilized more proficiently, yielding an efficient delivery of care, and empowering residents and their significant others to become an active partner in their own care. Once the culture is transitioned, it will become an important factor to the continuous quality improvement efforts of the facility.

Building the Team

To build an interdisciplinary team, you need to begin by choosing team members who are qualified and motivated to work toward a better dementia care program. Members must believe that the mission to develop a quality dementia care program is important to the quality of life of the residents. Discipline-specific members represented on the team are dependent on the topic. For dementia care, the core team should include the following:

- Nursing team member
- Social services
- Activities team member
- Pharmacist
- Therapist
- Physician
- Dietary team member
- Charge nurse
- Nursing assistant

Team Management

In preparation for effective team management, it will be important to meet the core learning needs of the team and clarify expectations. These include:
- Organize regular meeting times, stressing the importance of timeliness and participation.
- Articulate roles and responsibilities.
- Set standards for team behavior.
- Develop effective communication strategies during and in between meetings.
- Establish common goals.
- Assess team efficacy and make changes accordingly.
- Train on conflict management and creative problem solving. Conflict is inevitable and may even encourage successful resolution of differences, resulting in a more cohesive team.

Sources of Conflict

Healthy sources of conflict include:
- Differences in opinion
- Variances in expectations
- Personality differences
- Differentiation in skill
- Different education levels

Unhealthy sources of conflict include:
- Hierarchy of positions
- Faulty communication
- Poor management
- Hidden agendas
- Competition over power

Conflict Resolution

Team conflict is inevitable. At first, there may not be any conflict since most individuals are usually polite during the initial stage of team building. However, as time passes and the team focuses on the project, conflicts may begin to surface regarding how to accomplish a task. Toward the end of the project, there is usually minimal conflict because each team member is focused on implementing the steps to accomplish the goals. This process is considered a natural part of team building, and with proper management, conflict can be constructive and may lead to a stronger team.

Each team member must appreciate and understand varying viewpoints. These viewpoints must be acknowledged and discussed with team members who will commit to reaching an agreement. Most conflict can be avoided by practicing active listening skills. Active listening involves employing the following skills:

- Not letting the message get personal
- Placing no blame
- Focusing on the task at hand

It is important and necessary to keep in mind that not all conflicts can be resolved to every team member's satisfaction.

The Facilitator's Role in Team Motivation

A loss in motivation can slow any team's progress toward their goals. The facilitator must remain attentive to any signs of a faltering team member. Loss of purpose or loss of ownership can occur when unrealistic goals are made. Clear and consistent goals will motivate the team if a reasonable timeline for progress and completion are set and reviewed on a regular basis. It is vital to acknowledge the progress and encourage the team to communicate continuing needs. It is also helpful to understand what drives each team member. A proactive and respectful facilitator will acknowledge the team's efforts and maintain the team members' engagement level. As a result, the team will be highly functional and the dementia care program will be successful at improving the quality of life and quality of care of residents.

Chapter 4: Conditions That Impact Cognitive Functioning

There are several conditions that can impact cognitive function and may co-exist with dementia, which can make it more difficult to manage behavioral symptoms. Healthcare professionals must understand the negative consequences, such as behavior disturbances, when these conditions are unidentified or mismanaged. Common conditions associated with dementia and possible contributory factors include the following below.

Decline in physical function can result from the following conditions:
- Pain
- Lack of resident participation in activities of daily living
- Poor nutrition, poor hydration
- Emerging acute condition
- Not recovered from recent acute condition

Sleep disturbances can result from the following conditions:
- Pain
- Nocturia
- Visual misperceptions
- Noise levels
- Room temperature
- Early rising
- Emerging acute condition
- Not recovered from acute condition
- Delirium

Fatigue can result from the following conditions:
- Lack of task segmentation
- Complex tasks too late in the day
- Poly-pharmacy
- Poor nutrition, poor hydration
- Hormonal imbalances
- Emerging acute condition
- Not recovered from acute condition

Anxiety and agitation can result from the following conditions:
- Lack of task segmentation
- Noise levels
- Too-large activity groups
- Environmental overstimulation
- Toileting needs
- Hunger
- Fatigue
- Emerging acute condition
- Not recovered from acute condition
- Staff not explaining procedure before care delivery

- Misinterpretation of the event
- Delirium

Depression can result from the following conditions:
- Lack of person-centered interests
- Pain
- Unable to communicate causing lack of socialization
- Hearing problems
- Vision problems

Poor appetite can result from the following conditions:
- Pain
- Poor vision
- Lack of person-centered food preferences
- Poly-pharmacy
- Impending acute condition
- Not recovered from acute condition

Cognitive declines and behaviors do not affect everyone equally, and each of us will most likely develop some degree of cognitive decline to one degree or another in our lifetime. Our ability to think and reason will affect how we respond to our environment and our physical conditions.

Behaviors are not only challenging for caregivers, they are distressing both physically and psychologically to the person with dementia. Emotional or physical distress can negatively impact their health and quality of life. The severity of the behavior, when physiological and psychological needs are not met, can also attribute to the risk of physical injury.

While most brain changes that occur with dementia are irreversible and worsen over time, treatable conditions may exacerbate the dementia behaviors. The result is a behavior that becomes the primary method of the resident's non-verbal expression. Our responsibility is to identify and address the reversible conditions and factors causing the distressed behavior. Identifying and addressing the underlying cause of the treatable condition may improve overall behavior, improve quality of life, and help preserve the dignity of residents.

Chapter 5: Assessment of Behavioral Conditions

Strengthening the assessment of behavioral conditions is a priority before implementing any potential interventions. One must understand the type of dementia the resident has, the purpose of the behavior, and conduct a thorough root cause analysis in order to promote a person-centered approach.

It is helpful to begin by distinguishing between the "3 D's": dementia, delirium, and depression in order to determine the physiological cause of the behavior. When we identify other reasons for behavior symptoms, this process is called "determining differential diagnosis." This is because not all cognitive deficits are contributed to dementia and may be reversible.

Dementia

Dementia is insidious and progresses over months or years. Alertness is usually normal, but orientation will deteriorate as the dementia gradually progresses. The resident may attempt to answer questions but will not be aware of mistakes, and there will be an inability to learn new information or to recall previously learned information. For most types of dementia, short-term memory fails first, and then long-term memory becomes more impaired as time goes on. The resident will be confused, and commonly with Parkinson's dementia, delusions are present. Perception is typically normal until the later stages. Irritability advances with the progression of dementia. Sleep patterns become irregular due to the disorientation to time. Dementia is difficult to diagnose early on since mini-mental exam scores may be high even with obvious cognitive impairment. For this reason, additional detailed tests are necessary. More detailed testing includes history and physical, neurological exam, physical exam, CT scan, and MRI. Additional testing may include laboratory testing to determine the status of electrolytes, blood count, liver function, calcium, B12, folate, thyroid, HIV, and include a urine examination. While the progression can be slightly decelerated with medication, it cannot be reversed.

Delirium

Delirium is a rapid-onset acute organic condition, and alertness may fluctuate and last for hours, days, or weeks. It will be difficult to engage the resident due to the orientation impairment and confusion. At times, the resident may become suspicious and suffer from hallucinations or delusions. As the resident continues to misinterpret the environment, he or she may become agitated or withdrawn. Sleep patterns are also irregular due to confusion. Nursing assistants should communicate any subtle changes in condition as soon as possible to the nurse so that the underlying condition can be addressed by the nurse with the physician immediately. Delirium is a result of medical, social, or environmental conditions, and early recognition is the key to keeping the resident safe.

Depression

Depression is a variable condition that may last for weeks or months. Orientation is usually normal but short-term memory may be impaired. Often, there is a preoccupation with negative ideation and the thought process may appear to be diminished. Delusions with a flat affect are present and the resident will exhibit irritability. Sleep patterns are disturbed resulting from confusion. Some residents will deny being depressed and exhibit increased complaints of physical illnesses, and staff may observe episodes of anxiety and social withdrawal.

Root Cause Analysis

If the behaviors are due to dementia, we can conduct a root cause analysis to identify exactly what the resident is trying to communicate, or trying to accomplish. If the behavior is due to delirium, we know that there is an underlying acute condition that needs our attention. And, if the behavior is due to depression, we know that we cannot accurately assess cognitive status until the depression is addressed.

As previously discussed, there are several types of dementia. Distinguishing between the characteristics for each of them, to obtain a diagnosis, is challenging. For example, there are clinical criteria overlap for Alzheimer's dementia, Lewy body dementia, and Parkinson's disease. For this reason, it is important to note that a formal diagnosis of dementia be obtained by a medical specialist such as a geriatrician, neurologist, or psychologist. Many times, physicians may choose to conduct these assessments on admission to the nursing home to establish a baseline for future comparison, and also to identify additional conditions that can be improved. The chart below, as depicted by the American Medical Directors Association (AMDA) *Dementia in the Long Term Care Setting– Clinical Practice Guideline*, depicts the differences between these dementias (Table 5.1).

Table 5.1 Differences between dementias

Characteristic	Alzheimer's disease dementia	Lewy Body dementia	Parkinson's disease dementia
Course of the disease	Gradual	Fluctuating	Gradual
Initial presentation	Dementia	Dementia, extrapyramidal symptoms	Extrapyramidal symptoms
Cognitive symptoms	Progressive from disease onset	Onset of dementia within one year of motor symptoms	Dementia usually occurs more than two years after extrapyramidal symptoms
Psychosis	Delusions more often than hallucinations	Visual hallucinations. Hallucinations are what usually distinguishes Lewy body from other dementias.	Medication-induced visual hallucinations more common
Motor symptoms	Gait disturbances and rigidity in later stages only	Bradykinesia, rigidity, gait disturbance, intention tremor	Resting tremor, rigidity, bradykinesia, postural imbalance

Table 5.1: Differences between dementias (cont.)

Hypersensitivity to antipsychotics	No	Yes	Yes
Neuropathology: Protein	Beta amyloid plaques between nerve synapses	Cortical and brain stem Lewy bodies, beta amyloid plaques between nerve synapses, alpha synucleinopathy	Brain stem Lewy bodies, alpha synucleinopathy

Once the type of dementia is determined, and the root cause of the behavior identified, the dementia care team can begin to implement person-centered interventions. The triggers to behaviors can often be identified by asking the following questions:

- What was the resident trying to do when the behavior occurred?
- What happened just before the behavior occurred?
- What makes the behavior better, and what makes it worse?
- Did the behavior follow a change in environment?
- Was there another individual near the resident just prior, or at the time of behavior?
- Did the behavior follow a specific event?
- Are there any subtle signs or symptoms to an impending acute condition?
- Has the resident experienced a recent acute condition?
- Is there a history of the same type of behavior?
- What is the impact of this specific behavior on other people?

A successful dementia care program is dependent on accurate diagnosis and interventions targeted to the root cause of the behavior. Establishing a baseline on admission is recommended to more accurately identify changes in condition later on during the episode of care. Continuous monitoring and adjusting approaches as needed will ensure that the resident's behavioral condition will improve, resulting in optimum functioning and a better quality of life.

Chapter 6: Non-Pharmacological Approaches to Managing Dementia Behaviors

When behavioral or psychological symptoms of dementia are exhibited, it means that during the course of the disease the resident will have an altered thought process, with difficulty integrating and retrieving new information. Non-pharmacological methods to address the behavior are the best initial approach, unless it is an emergency situation, once the identifiable cause for the behavior is determined.

Medications used for the purpose of managing behaviors that have no identifiable cause are likely to be ineffective, and can result in complications such as falls, fractures, cerebral-vascular events, and even death. The U.S. Food and Drug Administration provides black box warnings for atypical antipsychotics, which indicate an increased risk of death when used for dementia-related psychosis. For these reasons, preparing an interdisciplinary behavior care plan with non-pharmacological interventions that capitalize on the resident's remaining strengths may decrease the use of unnecessary medications.

Non-Pharmacological Considerations

Repetitive speech, sleep disturbances, and wandering are common core features of Alzheimer's disease and related dementias. Targeting approaches to the resident's current cognitive function, physical function, spiritual well-being, and revising interventions as necessary will optimize quality of life. The following chart lists non-pharmacological considerations for specific behaviors (Table 6.1).

Table 6.1: Non-pharmacological considerations for specific behaviors

Behavior	Consideration
Resisting care	Evaluate pain status
	Evaluate sleep patterns
	Provide positive distraction
	Provide consistent caregivers
	Personalize environment
	Allow time to process instructions
	Evaluate vision and hearing
	Provide simple cues

Table 6.1: Non-pharmacological considerations for specific behaviors (cont.)

Disruptive in group activities	Determine whether toileting needs exist
	Provide rest periods
	Provide small group activities
	Provide activities that are broken into simple steps
	Provide snacks and refreshments
	Offer activities of preferences and interests or that are related to previous occupation
	Offer activities to promote calmness, such as slow tapping, drumming, clapping, rocking, or swinging
Verbally or physically abusive	Provide companionship
	Develop trust
	Avoid confrontation
	Provide massage or touch therapy
	Redirect to desirable activity or familiar activities (folding, sorting, matching)
	Decrease external stimuli
	Identify trigger and avoid trigger
	Provide favorite snack
	Review familiar photographs
Rummaging	Provide normalizing activities (sorting socks, folding towels)
	Provide rummaging areas such as dressers, purses, boxes
	Use "no entry" cues such as "do not disturb" signs

Table 6.1: Non-pharmacological considerations for specific behaviors (cont.)

Sudden mood changes	Assess for impending acute condition
	Evaluate pain status
	Assess for hyperglycemia and hypoglycemia
	Accommodate customary schedule
	Provide consistent routines
	Provide consistent caregivers
	Decrease noise levels
Withdrawing from previous interests	Provide activities just before or after meals where meals are served
	Provide in-room visits
	Invite resident to special events
	Engage in activities that emphasize personal history and knowledge
Wandering/elopement risk	Take resident for a walk
	Provide distraction of preferred activity
	Alleviate fears
	Provide space and environmental cues to reduce exit behavior (seating along walking path, objects to manipulate along the walking path, room with calm setting, rocking chairs, music)
	Aroma therapy
	Initiate conversations about what they are seeking
	One-on-one activities during active wandering times
	Provide pre-meal and post-meal activities
	Provide for toileting needs
	Provide room identifiers

Behaviors are usually how a person with dementia communicates an unmet need. Staff must respond with a calm, non-judgmental approach. Observations on what happened before and after the behavior occurred could help identify the trigger, which may include physical comfort, sense of competency, need for socialization, or the desire to communicate effectively.

Communication

The resident or family representative must be involved, to the extent possible, in the care planning process with an interdisciplinary goal to prevent or reduce targeted behaviors. Educating staff and family members on effective communication strategies can enhance non-pharmacological interventions. Communication strategies include using a calm voice, offering no more than two choices, avoid open-ended questions, keeping discussions and questions simple, relaxing activity rules so that the resident will not feel they are performing inadequately, and using cues to initiate and execute daily activities.

Chapter 7: Pharmacological Approaches to Managing Dementia Behaviors

It is important to recognize that in 2014, the National Partnership to Improve Dementia Care succeeded in reducing antipsychotic use by 15.1% across the United States. However, there are other issues related to a comprehensive dementia care program that still require improvement. These issues include:

- Improving pain management
- Improving the decision-making process
- Reducing caregiver stress
- Improving assessment of dementia care practices
- Working toward antipsychotic reduction

Using Medication in Dementia Care Programs

Behaviors or psychological symptoms of dementia (BPSD) such as depression, agitation, wandering, and delusions are common in the moderate-to-severe stages of dementia. Non-pharmacological approaches are the first alternative to medications for the treatment of BPSD, as are avoiding the use of physical or chemical restraints, except in emergency situations. Many classes of medication, including antipsychotics, antidepressants, and anticonvulsants have been used off-label to treat these behaviors. Of all of these, antipsychotics have been utilized most often due to their proven benefit in short-term use. Antipsychotic medications should be used only after the following causes have been ruled out:

- Medical
- Physical
- Functional
- Psychological
- Emotional
- Psychiatric
- Social
- Environmental

Both first generation (typical) and second generation (atypical) antipsychotics are associated with increased mortality when used for BPSD in the elderly, and the care team should be aware that the use of antipsychotics can contribute to falls, weight loss, infection, and incontinence. Because of this, the lowest possible dose with the shortest period of time should be used when antipsychotics are prescribed, and gradual dosage reduction, unless contraindicated, is necessary.

Antipsychotics for those with dementia should not be used if the only indications are for the following:
- Wandering
- Restlessness
- Impaired memory
- Mild anxiety
- Insomnia
- Refusal of care

While the use of antipsychotics may possibly be appropriate at times, the diagnosis alone does not warrant its use unless the following criteria are also met:

1. The behavior symptoms pose a danger to the resident or others, and
2. One or both of the following:
    - The symptoms are due to mania or psychosis, such as auditory, visual, or other hallucinations; delusions, paranoia, or grandiosity;
    - Behavioral interventions have been attempted and included in the plan of care, except in an emergency

Emergency Use of Antipsychotics

Antipsychotic use warrants additional criteria when initiated or used to treat an emergency situation. Emergency use must be related to an acute onset or exacerbation of symptoms or immediate threats to the health and safety of the resident or others. In addition, all of the following requirements must be met:

1. Acute treatment period limited to seven days or less.
2. A clinician, along with the interdisciplinary team, must evaluate and document the emergency situation within seven days. Contributing factors and underlying causes of the acute condition must be included in this documentation.

3. If behaviors persist beyond the emergency situation, non-pharmacological interventions must be attempted, unless clinically contraindicated. These interventions must be documented following the resolution of the acute event.

Enduring Conditions and Antipsychotic Use

Before initiating or increasing a dosage for antipsychotic medication, monitoring is necessary to ensure the behavioral symptoms are:

1. Not due to a medical condition that is expected to improve or resolve when the underlying condition is treated
2. Not due to environmental stressors that can be addressed to improve the symptoms
3. Not due to psychological stressors (abuse, anxiety, fear, loneliness) stemming from a cognitive impairment that is expected to improve or resolve once the situation is addressed
4. Persistent behaviors, documented in the medial record, that the condition recurs over time or continues with documented prior approaches that failed to manage the symptom

New Admissions

When a new admission arrives with antipsychotic medication orders, the facility is still responsible for the following:

- Preadmission screening (PASSR)
- Orders for care that include appropriate clinical indications for the use of the antipsychotic medication

For those residents who do not require a PASSR and have orders for antipsychotic medication, the facility must reevaluate its use on admission or within two weeks of admission (at the time of the initial Minimum Data Set assessment) to consider whether the medication can be reduced or discontinued.

Risks vs. Benefits of Antipsychotic Use

When a resident is prescribed antipsychotics, adequate monitoring must take place to look for signs and symptoms of adverse consequences. These consequences may include:

- Anticholinergic effects (falls, sedation)
- Cardiovascular (arrhythmias, orthostatic hypotension)
- Metabolic (poorly controlled blood glucose level)
- Weight gain
- Increase in cholesterol and triglycerides
- Neurological symptoms (parkinsonism, ardive dyskinesia, stroke, transient ischemic attack, akathisia)

When the antipsychotic medication causes or contributes to these problems, an evaluation of the medication use must be completed to determine whether the benefits still outweigh the risks. If it is determined the benefit outweighs the risk, the prescriber must document the rationale for the decision to continue the antipsychotic medication. In addition, the resident or the resident's representative must be aware of the benefits and risks, and involved in the decision-making process.

Chapter 8: Monitoring Outcomes of Approaches

To monitor the outcomes of dementia care approaches, first it is necessary to assess the underlying cause of the problem. The problem may be a behavioral or psychological symptom of dementia, or it could be an underlying treatable condition that is causing a specific behavior. In both cases, it is necessary to identify all of the factors that contribute to the root cause of the problem and analyze its impact on physical, mental, and psychosocial needs of the resident. This process is called root cause analysis and will also focus on whether the symptom or condition impacts the function, mood, or cognition of the resident before determining that the behavior is an actual problem. Once the root cause is identified, you should begin the PDSA cycle (Plan, Do, Study, Act). The PDSA cycle is a systematic four-step process for performance improvement. It can be used to address multiple issues and problems at all levels of the facility, and the dementia care team will use it to address resident-specific problems. While root cause analysis will address assessment and underlying cause identification, the PDSA cycle will continue to target the problem by addressing elements of the surveyor guidance to dementia care, which include care planning, implementation of the care plan, care plan revisions, and monitoring.

Plan

Plan the intervention to target the root cause of the problem and determine whether the cognitive patterns, mood, and behavior present a risk to the resident or others. If the problem has the potential to pose a risk, then the dementia care team, which includes the resident or resident's representative and the physician, will collaborate on setting an outcome goal that is realistic to achieve. Consider prior life patterns and preferences when setting the goal.

Do

Implement the interventions to the plan according to the resident's wishes and current standards of practice. Document the interventions and communicate the target behaviors and interventions to frontline staff. Ensure that there is a sufficient number of staff on duty to carry out the plan.

Study

Analyze the outcome of the interventions to evaluate whether the goals were met. Reassess the effectiveness of the plan with input from the resident or resident's representative, and staff, ensuring the interventions supported the resident's highest practicable level of physical, mental, and psychosocial well-being.

Act

Act on the findings, modifying interventions as necessary. If the goal was not met, determine the reason, revise approaches, and re-set the goal. If the goal was attained, the dementia care team will determine whether the current interventions will be continued or change.

Quality Assessment and Assurance

Facility procedures must clearly outline a systematic process for dementia care. The Quality Assessment and Assurance committee (QAA) and the Quality Assurance Performance Improvement (QAPI) committee must monitor for consistent implementation of the policy and procedures. Monitoring and oversight for dementia care is everyone's responsibility, with the chairperson of the QAA and QAPI committee providing education and resources (dementia experts, medical specialists, facilitators, staff, etc.) to provide a successful dementia care program.

Monitoring Outcomes of Non-Pharmacological and Pharmacological Approaches

In both instances, an evaluation of the interventions and their impact on the target behaviors should be conducted at the following times:

- At the conclusion of the PDSA cycle
- At every Minimum Data Set (MDS) completion
- With any new antipsychotic medication or dosage change
- With every change in condition
- With emergence of new behaviors
- With the worsening of behaviors

Some facilities may choose to utilize behavior-monitoring logs. When logs are utilized, each target behavior must be listed separately with specific interventions. Simply documenting that the behavior has occurred is not sufficient. Each time the targeted behavior occurs, the documentation must indicate which intervention was utilized and the outcome of the intervention. Questions to determine the efficacy of the interventions include:

- Has the behavior decreased in occurrence or severity?
- Is the resident experiencing less distress?
- Have the interventions optimized resident function?
- If medication is used to manage the behavior, is the resident experiencing any side effects of the medication? If side effects are present, the medication dosage should be adjusted, or the medication should be changed or discontinued.
- If medication was utilized, did the team discuss the risks versus the benefits?
- If medication was utilized, were timely reductions attempted?
- If medication is not tapered, is there thorough risk versus benefit documentation by the physician in the medical record?
- At each review (MDS completion, new antipsychotic medication orders or dosage changes, every change in condition, emergence of new behaviors, worsening of behaviors), are all the current interventions still necessary?

Monitoring the Efficacy of Interventions

Monitoring the efficacy of interventions for dementia symptoms and its complications will prevent further functional declines. Interventions must be individualized, based on the appropriate assessment of the behavioral symptoms, and consistent. Staff must continuously respond appropriately to the changing needs of dementia residents in order to optimize function and quality of life while utilizing non-pharmacological approaches, when safe and feasible.

Chapter 9: Dementia Care and Activities Staff

From restraint reduction to reducing unnecessary medications, activity professionals will encounter multiple opportunities to contribute with person-centered approaches to dementia care. Too often facilities do not investigate the root cause of the dementia behavior symptoms, resulting in approaches that are ineffective. Boredom, meaningless activities, loneliness, and helplessness can contribute to distressing behaviors. With a collaborative interdisciplinary approach, providing meaningful activities as an approach to managing dementia symptoms can decrease distressing dementia behaviors and result in the elimination of inappropriate restraint use and reducing or eliminating the need for antipsychotic medication, promoting dignity and safety for residents.

The long-term care *State Operations Manual, Appendix PP* regulatory tag number F248, defines an activity program as any endeavor, other than routine activities of daily living, that is intended to enhance a sense of well-being and to promote or enhance physical, cognitive, and emotional health. It also states that the facility will identify each resident's interests and needs, involve the resident in an ongoing program of activities that is designed to appeal to his or her interests, and enhances the resident's highest practicable level of physical, mental, and psychosocial well-being. These are important concepts in dementia care and should be at the forefront of every dementia care program.

Whether the facility functions with a traditional approach of a centralized activity department, or a nontraditional household model with all staff providing activities that reflect daily life (preparing foods, chores, etc.), the regulatory expectation remains the same for both.

Dementia Care Activity Considerations

Utilizing multiple sources (observations of when the behavior occurs, interviews with staff on what precipitates the behavior, the MDS assessment) the dementia care activity will be developed to match the skills, abilities, needs, and preferences of the resident. These activities must be consistent with the resident's cognitive and physical ability, providing assistance and approaches to enable the resident to be engaged to the best of his or her ability.

The interdisciplinary team must keep in mind that medications such as diuretics resulting in toileting needs, or conditions such as pain, can influence participation in the activities attempted. Other types of situations may also interfere with the success of the activities such as hearing impairments, vision impairments, or fatigue, which may exacerbate dementia behaviors during an activity. The resident with dementia may not be able to communicate these needs, so the crucial consideration is to approach every dementia care activity situation collaboratively to determine what is interfering with the success of the activity, otherwise the result may be unnecessary restraint or antipsychotic use.

Activities and Approaches to Specific Behavior Symptoms

Once the specific behavior symptoms are identified, the interdisciplinary team can collaborate on the best approaches. Minimizing specific dementia behavior symptoms may include, but are not limited to, the following suggestions (Table 9.1):

Table 9.1: Suggestions for minimizing specific dementia behavior symptoms

Constantly walking	• Provide an environment with seating areas along a walking path that includes objects that the resident can stop and manipulate
	• Provide a room with a calming atmosphere that includes music, lighting, and rocking chairs (e.g., Snoezelen therapy room, massage room)
	• Engage the resident in conversation about what he or she is seeking or looking for
Hitting, yelling, or other compulsive behavior	• Provide a calm environment with structured activities such as sorting, folding, and matching
	• Use small group activities
	• Provide a favorite snack

Table 9.1: Suggestions for minimizing specific dementia behavior symptoms (cont.)

Disruptive demanding behaviors or catastrophic reactions such as crying or anger	• Provide achievable activities in small, simple steps • Use small group activities • Use short and repetitive activities that can be stopped if the resident becomes overwhelmed • Involve the resident in familiar activities such as occupation-related tasks • Utilize slow exercises such as tapping and drumming
Going through other's belongings	• Provide activities that include sorting, stacking, or other organizational tasks • Provide rummaging areas in plain sight that include dressers or a chest of drawers with clothing or other items • Place removable "Do not disturb" signs for those residents' doors whose rooms are being rummaged

Table 9.1: Suggestions for minimizing specific dementia behavior symptoms (cont.)

Withdrawing from previous activity	• Provide an activity outside of the room just before or after where meals are being served • Invite the resident to activities and be accompanied by a trusted family member • Provide opportunities to participate in activities that emphasize the resident's history such as a sport or cultural activity • Plan an activity outdoors
Lacking personal safety awareness that causes injury or potential injury to self	• Involve in smaller group activities • Use activities that are soothing such as music or talking about personal skills (e.g., baking, gardening)
Exhibiting delusions or hallucinations	• Focus on familiar activities and provide verbal reassurance to decrease stress and improve awareness of actual surroundings

During a survey, staff will be expected to identify which approaches are used to address specific behaviors. A periodic review at the time of an MDS assessment, at every change in condition, and with every new behavior symptom must be completed to identify any adjustments needed to previous approaches. All staff should commit to every approach being designed to engage the resident in life, which means that the events listed on the standard activity calendar may not be appropriate for all residents with dementia behavioral symptoms. Staff members providing activities to residents with dementia should focus on the following items:

- Increase pleasant and desirable experiences for the resident.
- Assist the resident to achieve his or her highest potential for participation in activities.
- Encourage the expression of thoughts, memories, and using all five senses throughout the day (sight, smell, hearing, taste, touch).
- Recognize early signs and triggers of agitation to avoid a negative event.
- Utilize communication, validation, and distraction techniques when necessary
- Be aware of communication perceptions such as body language, gestures, facial expressions, and tone of voice.
- Be aware that approaches may change as the dementia progresses.
- Avoid making assumptions. A diagnosis of dementia does not automatically negate that the resident can participate in activities at one level or another.

The Dementia Care Team Focus

During dementia care team meetings, time should be set aside to discuss the effectiveness of approaches and to share creative ideas to further support the resident with dementia and to identify staff training needs. Above all else, staff members who perform activities for those with dementia must be creative, exhibit patience, and believe that participation in meaningful activities is possible.

Dementia Care Resources

Advancing Excellence in America's Nursing Homes

The Advancing Excellence Campaign provides tools and resources to improve nursing homecare.

www.nhqualitycampaign.org

The Alzheimer's Association

The Alzheimer's Association is the world's leading voluntary health organization in Alzheimer's care, support, and research. It provides information on dementia symptoms, diagnosis, stages, treatment, care, and support resources. Its mission is to eliminate Alzheimer's disease through the advancement of research; to provide and enhance care and support to all affected; and to reduce the risk of dementia through the promotion of brain health.

www.alz.org

Carmelina: Essential Nursing Systems for Long-Term Care

This resource manual follows Carmelina, a fictional character, through her nursing home experience. Case studies, which can be used for staff education, demonstrate how to build solid nursing systems and how person-centered care can improve quality of life.
http://traininginmotion.org/CARMELINA.html

CMS *Hand-In-Hand Toolkit*

CMS provides a training series for dementia care and abuse prevention. The mission of the Hand-In-Hand training is to provide nursing homes with a high-quality training program that emphasizes person-centered care for those with dementia.
www.cms-handinhandtoolkit.info

Dementia Care: The Quality Chasm, January 2013

From the Dementia Initiative group, this white paper was developed from a number of sources and discusses person-centered dementia care, including barriers and challenges to dementia care delivery.
www.leadingage.org/Dementia_Care_CCAL_Whitepaper.aspx

Dementia in the Long Term Care Setting Clinical Practice Guideline

From the American Medical Directors Association (AMDA), it is one of several guidelines undertaken by AMDA's mission to improve quality of care for nursing home residents. It includes chapters on recognition, assessment, treatment, and monitoring.
www.amda.com/tools/guidelines.cfm#dementia

Implementing Change in Long-Term Care: A Practical Guide to Transformation

This resource was prepared with a grant from the Commonwealth Fund to the Pioneer Network. It is a resource for implementing culture change (not Quality Assurance and Performance Improvement [QAPI]), and it is a good resource on the change process.
www.pioneernetwork.net/Data/Documents/Implementation_Manual_ChangeInLongTermCare%5B1%5D.pdf

INTERACT II

INTERACT II is a system of tools to improve communication on change in condition. This comprehensive set of tools may be considered part of a QAPI process toolkit.
www.interact2.net

Quality Improvement Organizations

Each state's Quality Improvement Organization (QIO) offers resources and tools for nursing homes. Many system tools are available free of charge. Once on the site, go to Quality Improvement, then the QIO Directory to search for tools at each QIO.
www.qualitynet.org

State Operations Manual, Appendix PP, F309 and F329

The *State Operations Manual* gives the state survey agency guidance to review care and services for a resident with dementia. It is a comprehensive resource for ensuring quality dementia care that includes a review of assessment, cause identification, care planning, implementation of the care plan, care plan revisions, and quality assessment and assurance.

World Alzheimer Report 2013: *Journey of Caring: An analysis of long-term care for dementia*

This report examines the latest regional and global trends of dementia care, and analyzes long-term care systems around the world.
www.alz.co.uk/research/world-report-2013

Note: URLs listed were current as of the date of this publication. HCPro is not responsible for the content or accessibility of these sites, nor implies endorsement.